"The non-diet diet book, Food for Thought is a straightforward, truly personalized approach to weight management. Ms. Cox invites the reader to understand who they are, choices to make, and the benefits of successfully managing food in our lives."

—Tom Doolittle, PhD, Licensed Clinical Psychologist

"Susan Cox's book reflects a practical approach to weight management. My patients experienced successful weight loss by following the common sense guidelines in Food for Thought."

—Dr. Marc Boyd, Boyd Obstetrics and Gynecology, Peoria Illinois

"The 'less is more mentality' of Food for Thought is a breath of fresh air within today's confusing and complex diet industry milieu. Susan Cox's advice for healthful eating is practical, simple, and 'right-on'. Ms. Cox provides suggestions that offer benefits not just in the short-term, but for a lifetime."

—Catherine A. Peterson, PhD, RD, Department of Nutritional Sciences, University of Missouri-Columbia

Food for Thought

Food for Thought

❖

A Menu of How to Eat and Live in Good Health

Susan M. Cox, RD

iUniverse, Inc.
New York Lincoln Shanghai

Food for Thought
A Menu of How to Eat and Live in Good Health

iUniverse, Inc.

For information address:
iUniverse, Inc.
2021 Pine Lake Road, Suite 100
Lincoln, NE 68512
www.iuniverse.com

ISBN: 0-595-30972-0

Printed in the United States of America

Contents

Author's Note

Anyone can call himself a "nutritionist." Many people are unaware that the title "nutritionist" can be used by anyone regardless of their educational background. No formal nutritional training or degree is required to accompany this often-misused title. A celebrity, a doctor, a pharmacist, or a plumber can all call themselves a "nutrition expert" or a "nutritionist" without ever having read or studied a single nutritional fact. Registered dietitians, on the other hand, must have a bachelor's of science degree in nutrition from an accredited university. Following graduation, they must pass a registration exam. They must then maintain specific continued education credits in order to keep their registration certificate current.

I am a registered dietitian. More importantly, I am a registered dietitian with clinical experience in weight management. I have real life, practical, personal experience with food issues, and I have successfully counseled many clients in managing their individual food issues. I know how to eat and live in good health, and I can teach you how to eat and live in good health.

Obesity is a serious issue in America. Research has shown that excessive weight gain increases your risk of developing life-threatening illnesses including heart disease, stroke, diabetes, cancer, and high blood pressure. Because obesity is such a serious issue, there are literally thousands of diet books and health and fitness magazines addressing weight control. Some are written by "nutritionists." Others are written by the most popular celebrity claiming to be a "nutrition expert." Books that are written by certain medical professionals may have adequate nutritional information, but what works in the lab isn't always applicable to people's real lives. I believe that people are fed up with fad diets, quick fixes, and magic pills that just don't work. People are tired of spending their hard-earned money on diet books with complicated food plans and confusing biochemical and nutritional terminology. They are frustrated with spending precious time sifting through the latest health and fitness magazines for that one tip that might work for them. A successful approach to weight control must be straightforward and concise.

Food for Thought contains all the information you will ever need for successful weight loss, in one simple, easy to read book. *Food for Thought* is not a diet plan. It is not another diet book filled with page after page of technical nutritional terms. It does not contain complicated, unrealistic food choices and planned eating schedules. Instead, *Food for Thought* recognizes that every person has individual nutritional needs based on their genetics, gender, activity level, and lifestyle behaviors. One diet plan will not work for everyone. *Food for Thought* will teach you how to make your own nutritional and fitness decisions. It was written to inspire you, the reader, to take control of your own health and fitness issues.

Food for Thought is the first, last, and only book you will ever need to help you with weight management. It is an easy, practical, and personal approach towards weight control. *Food for Thought* will help you acquire the knowledge and confidence you need to live a healthy, productive life. It is time to give yourself some serious food for thought!

Dig in and Bon Appétit!

Acknowledgements

I wish to thank the following people who encouraged me to share my knowledge and experience in nutrition and healthy living:

To my mom who always had time to read to me when I was little, and who quietly encouraged me to write this book.

To my dad who told me countless stories about the Grey Pony, and who always has a good joke to share.

To my husband, Brian, who has seen and believed in my talents even when they were hidden from me, myself, and I.

And to our girls, Corinne and Brenna, my little food snobs, may you always live your lives healthfully, happily, and to your greatest potential.

A special thanks to all of my siblings who always voted for me as mom's favorite at our family reunions!

A very special thank you to my friend, Barb Friedhoff, who suffered through the roughest of rough drafts of this book and had kind words to say anyway. And for coming up with the book title when creativity escaped me!

And my deepest gratitude to all of my clients who made the commitment to change their lifestyles and get healthy! It was an honor to share in your successes, and you are the true inspiration behind this book. Congratulations!

Preface

Her sisters would tease her as they playfully poked her tummy and said, "Dough-boy!" Just five years old, she was a shy little girl with light brown hair, blue eyes, spindly legs, and a belly that stuck out like Buddha's. That little round tummy always protruded from her too small hand-me-down-shirts. She knew her sisters were only joking, but the teasing hurt nonetheless.

The same little girl, ten years later, sat in a high school classroom. A girl in the seat next to her leaned over, laughed, and pointed, "Your stomach sticks out over your belt!" Inside, the girl was mortified, but she laughed off the comment and desperately tried to hold her stomach in for the rest of the day. Later that night, as she cried herself to sleep, she silently vowed that never again would anyone make fun of her body. She was not going to be a "fat little dough-boy" anymore.

That one day changed the girl forever. I know, because that girl was and is me. My lifelong issues with food began that day. My personal struggle with anorexia nervosa started there and it has taken great effort and perseverance to fight my food "demons" and to address my food issues. Still, I have come out on the other side and I am a smarter, stronger, and more compassionate person than I would have been had I not fought the battle.

It is through my personal struggle with anorexia, my recovery process, and my career choice in food and nutrition that I have come to realize that I am not alone in this journey. Each and every one of us has life experiences that may seem like small insignificant events, but those experiences shape us, and change us, and make us who we are. It is how we choose to use these experiences that is the ultimate challenge.

It is that challenge that has led me to write this book. I had a choice to keep my issues with food to myself, or to share my experiences and my nutritional education to help others who may have similar issues. I hope that this book will challenge you to explore your own personal issues that affect your eating patterns, and ultimately your life. We all have to eat to live. I hope to teach you how to eat and live healthfully, and more importantly, how to eat and live happily.

1

Life Issues

Issues with food, weight, and body image are not easy to talk about. Most people are looking for a quick fix, a magic pill, or the latest fad diet. But the reality is that there are no magic secrets or quick fix tips when it comes to managing your eating habits and maintaining a healthy weight. The only way to successfully manage your weight is through lifestyle changes. If you digest the food, exercise, and weight management tips found on the following pages, and apply these ideas and techniques to your daily life, you will successfully manage your weight. But, to do so, you must commit right now to wanting to make the necessary changes in your life in order to meet your personal weight goals. No excuses. No whining. I will cover the concepts of successful weight management, but you are ultimately the one who must do the work. And weight control is hard work. If it were easy, we wouldn't be a nation of people with serious weight and food issues, on the brink of a national health care disaster. The number one and two killers in the United States are heart disease and cancer. And what are they ultimately attributed to? You guessed it: the food we eat. The old adage, "you are what you eat," is not so far from the truth. If you eat junk, you are going to look bad and feel worse. If you eat healthy, you are going to look good and feel great!

I get a big kick out of people who take great pride in keeping their homes and cars and other material possessions in pristine condition, but these same people don't take care of their own health and bodies! Our homes and our cars need regular maintenance and occasional tune-ups. Well, our bodies deserve the same care and attention. You wouldn't put leaded gas into a car that calls for unleaded gas, would you? So why would you put unhealthy foods into a body that needs healthy food?

Healthy eating is really a very simple concept. If you read this book with an open mind regarding what food issues you may be struggling with, you will be successful in managing your personal weight issues. The information within these pages will guide you down the path to successful weight management and healthy food and exercise habits that will last you a lifetime.

I hope that this book will not become "just another diet book." There are as many diet books out there as there are dieters. Instead, I have tried to include nutritional tips and healthy eating advice that will get you thinking about what lifestyle changes will work for you as an individual. Look at this book as a menu, a feast of healthy living techniques that can help you enjoy food and enjoy life. This book will not teach you how to calculate your exact calorie needs or how to count fat grams. Frankly, I don't think the technique of counting anything works in the long run. The last thing that people who are obsessed with food need to do is to obsess about weighing and measuring food, or to spend time calculating fat grams or daily calories. This book will teach you how **not** to obsess about every little calorie and fat gram that you put into your mouth. But you will have some work to do in order to get healthy. You must be willing to be honest with yourself regarding the issues that you may have with your weight and with food in general. You must then be willing to use all of the information provided and carry through with the motivation to apply the information to your life. You will gain invaluable insight into yourself as an individual, and you will be amazed at your own abilities in regaining control over your weight and your life. And, maybe most importantly, you will be greatly relieved to learn that we all have issues! Let's get started and explore some food-related issues.

2

Weight and Body Image Issues

Everyone is an individual, and no one single diet therapy program works for everyone. Every person, who has been successful with long-term, weight management, has done so by following an individual food and exercise plan that works for them in their life situation. Some people may be able to handle having a bag of candy bars in their pantry; others may have to avoid having any candy at all in their homes because they can't resist the temptation. Some folks may enjoy biking as their favorite activity; others may focus on a brisk daily walk. That being said, every successful weight management program follows the same basic healthy guidelines, but these guidelines are tweaked and modified to fit into each individual's daily life plan. That is where you, as the individual, have to take responsibility and make the information in this book work for you.

Everyone has weight issues and other life issues! And I mean **everyone**! I don't care if you are a pencil-thin model, a "normal" weight twenty-year-old, or an overweight middle-aged frump. We all have weight issues. Don't judge that "perfect" size five mother of three any differently than you would judge her plus-size friend. They both have weight issues. The difference is in how they handle these "issues" on a daily basis. Let me clarify what I mean by weight issues, which is completely different from body size issues. The term "weight issues" refers to the struggle that each of us has every day in maintaining or achieving a desirable body weight. And let's face it; what is defined as a "desirable" weight is greatly influenced by society's definition of "The Perfect Body." I'm not saying that this is right or wrong, only that it is. The first and most important step in achieving your desirable weight, and dealing with your personal weight issues, is to be completely and totally honest with yourself regarding your body type. Otherwise, you are simply fighting a losing battle.

That brings me to the point of body shape. We are all largely (no pun intended) dependent on the genetic pool that determines whether we are well endowed on top, or carry our weight on the bottom half, or for that very small

Halle Berry percentage of the perfect gene pool, correctly proportioned from top to bottom. (Again, this is not to say that the Halle Berry types don't have "weight issues," only that they **appear** to manage them successfully.) But all of us can manage our weight and reach a desirable, and more importantly, healthy weight goal. The key to that statement is desirable and healthy. Some people are just not genetically meant to be a svelte perfect size five. It is not one perfect size or one specific number on the scale that we are trying to achieve here. What we are trying to achieve is a healthy body size and weight that fits you as an individual based on your genetic predisposition towards body shape. And by healthy, I mean healthy both physically and emotionally. If you spend all your time and energy trying to maintain a specific body weight, then you have completely lost sight of the concept of healthy living. The following is an example of what I mean by the misnomer "desirable" weight.

Find the best answer to the following question using the information provided.

A thirty-year-old woman is five feet three inches tall and weighs 140 pounds. Is she:

A.   Overweight

B.   At her target/desirable weight

C.   Neither of the above

NOTE: Use the following formula for "desirable" weight:

The formula for women: Give 100 pounds for the first five feet of height and add five pounds for every inch after five feet. (Example: A five foot one inch woman should weigh 105 pounds as her "desirable weight." You can add or subtract ten percent to this number to allow for body frame differences. This would give you a desirable body weight range of 94.5 pounds to 111.5 pounds.

The formula for men is: Give 106 pounds for the first five feet of height and six pounds for every inch after five feet. You may also add or subtract ten percent to this number to allow for body frame size differences.

The answer to the above question is (C). Why? Because even given the standard formula for "desirable" weight, you simply don't have enough information about the person to determine if she is overweight or not. Let me explain further. (A) would be the correct answer if this woman ate donuts and drank soda all day long as she sits on the couch reading diet and exercise books hoping to lose weight through osmosis. She would be consuming more calories than she burns off in a day's time. However, (B) would be your correct answer if this woman ran or walked three miles a day, read a chapter of this book every evening before bed, and did a good amount of weight training with heavy weights three to five times a week. She would carry more muscle mass on her body, and because muscle weighs more than fat, the scale would show a larger number but she would not be considered "overfat" or overweight. Therefore, (C) is the best answer because the numbers on the scale are not enough to determine whether someone is at a healthy fit weight for their height.

The moral of this lesson is two-fold. One, to be successful at long-term weight loss, you have to be honest with yourself and determine what your body shape is, and set reasonable and attainable weight loss goals for yourself. By the way, a safe and healthy weight loss goal is one to two pounds per week. If you lose weight any faster than that then you risk losing water or lean body tissue. And, your weight loss goals should change as you progress through the healthy lifestyle process. Secondly, don't sabotage yourself with daily weigh-in rituals. The scale should be used only as a basic guide and to check your progress once a week. If you weigh yourself once, or more than once a day, you only set yourself up for disappointment and defeat. Our bodies can fluctuate by three to five pounds a day (more if you are a larger person) just from a hydration standpoint. Water loss is not true weight loss. High protein diets promote unhealthy water weight loss and muscle loss.

3

Eating Out without Pigging Out

Let's tackle the issue of fast food. Did you know that the United States is the only developed country that has overweight people who are malnourished? An oxymoron you say? Not at all—think about it. We are a country that, for the most part, prides itself on the faster the food the better. Trust me on this one. I worked at fast food establishments as a teenager and we got timed on getting those orders out that drive-through window. The super-sized options are a whole other issue. Let's just say, if you order biggie fries, you're going to be a biggie person.

Fast foods and other convenience foods are by nature calorically dense and nutritionally lacking. In other words, they have, in general, a very high calorie and high fat content, but a very low vitamin and low mineral content. Therefore, we have a population of fast food/convenient food junkies who are potentially walking around with vitamin and mineral deficiencies. Let's consider the adolescent population as an example. Not only do they have vending machines at school providing them with unhealthy food and beverage options, but they also grab fast foods for dinner before rushing off to their extracurricular activities. It is simply easier to stop at a drive-through window than it is to take the time to pack a meal or snack. Plus, mom and dad don't have to worry about feeding the kids after a busy day at work. Eating out for teens is also extra social time with their friends. There are moments when I wonder if I am the only parent that sees the irony of pushing fast foods and junk foods at our kids as we chauffeur them around to their soccer, basketball, baseball, or dance practices. We have a whole population of kids who are getting way too many fat calories and total calories, but aren't getting enough nutrients for their growing bodies!

Calcium is a good example of a very common nutritional deficiency that can occur when soft drinks are consumed instead of milk. Milk is one of the best dietary sources of calcium. Osteoporosis is a chronic debilitating bone disease caused by long-term inadequate calcium intake. I won't bore you with statistical matter on this subject. There are numerous medical/nutritional journal articles to support these observations. My point is to make you aware that real vitamin and mineral deficiencies can and do occur when you substitute what we in the business refer to as "empty calorie" foods and beverages for healthier alternatives.

You may be wondering if the "diet" options at fast food restaurants are viable choices. Not in my book. Personally, I think most of the "diet" foods offered at these chains are simply taste bud suicide. Your choices range from a salad made with iceberg lettuce (no nutritional value) and diet (gag!) salad dressing, or the trendier yogurt parfaits, which come with calorically dense granola. (Low fat or not, granola is high in calories.) Or, there is the very weak attempt at nutritional consciousness with the veggie burger option at some chains. This would be an acceptable option **if** it were presented on a whole-wheat bun with mustard (negligible calories) and a nice dark green leaf of lettuce or two and a generous slice of tomato. So what is the bottom line with fast food if you want to be successful with long-term weight management? Simple. Just don't eat it. Ever. Period. Yes, the advice in this book is straight to the point, but not necessarily easy to swallow.

Let's move on to the subject of other sit-down restaurant options. You can eat out, occasionally. My rule of thumb with eating out at a non-fast food restaurant, is to limit it to once a week. Twice a week is pushing it. Most people enjoy a meal away from home every so often, sometimes, not even so much for the food, but for the simple pleasure of being waited on and not having to do the dishes!

Eating out can be a fun and enjoyable form of entertainment and needn't completely ruin your weight loss goals. The mantra to repeat when you dine out is simply "everything in moderation." Let me explain further. Restaurant portions are generally three to five times the normal portion size. Pasta selections can be up to seven times the normal portion size! Most people who have "dieted" are quite familiar with portion sizes. However, that being said, **knowing** what a normal portion size is and **eating** a normal portion size are two entirely different things. If you are unfamiliar with portion sizes, you can get information from the American Dietetic Association. Visit ADA's Web site at www.eatright.org. Familiarize yourself with the food pyramid to learn appropriate servings sizes.

Most people also know, at least in general, which menu items are the healthiest choices, but you may not always make those choices because you are "treating" yourself to a meal away from home. When counseling clients on weight control, quite often I find that many of my clients have a fairly good nutritional knowledge base, but they lack the skills to apply that information to their lives. Some people just need help getting motivated to follow a healthy eating plan. In fact, many of my clients are more knowledgeable about calorie and fat gram content than I am, but they don't follow through with applying those guidelines towards a healthy eating plan.

Therefore, I would like to review just a few things to keep in mind when ordering off the menu. First, it is perfectly acceptable to order a salad or an appetizer as your meal. If you do order an entrée, you can ask the waiter to serve you just half of your entrée, and to put the remainder in a doggie bag for you to take home. Out of sight, out of mind. Secondly, keep in mind that candlelight and dim lighting tend to lower your inhibitions and contribute to overeating. So be aware of your surroundings and how they can affect your mood. Just simply being aware of things that trigger you to eat more can help you avoid overeating in certain situations. Try to make healthy choices from the menu. In general, it is fairly easy to know which items are high fat, high calorie choices. For example, everyone knows fettuccini alfredo is a heart attack on a plate, and that a sixteen-ounce sirloin is going to do more damage than a petite fillet. And of course, any gravy, hollandaise, or cream sauce should be an automatic red flag! However, sometimes you may order what you believe to be a low fat, low calorie choice and it simply is not. Restaurants do not have to reveal how foods are prepared or what their calorie and fat content is. Don't be afraid to ask for your meal to be prepared without extra butter or oils. Some of the best chefs will admit that they will use pounds of butter to flavor favorite recipes!

A few restaurants are beginning to at least put symbols by some of their lower fat menu choices. Some restaurants refer to these choices as "heart healthy." There is a strong grass roots effort to get restaurants to provide nutritional information and to provide tasteful lower calorie menu choices and smaller serving sizes. However, it will take a lot more consumer support to become mainstream. If consumers keep buying the "biggie is more" logo, then that's what we'll continue to get. Also, keep in mind that high fat and high calorie need not be synonymous with great taste, especially in a restaurant where you have trained professional chefs preparing your meal. That is the best time to ask for or try lower fat menu choices because, the foods will be prepared by someone who knows how to do it using the freshest, most flavorful ingredients. This can be especially true when choosing vegetarian or spicy dishes. Learn to taste the actual food, not the oil or grease that's added to it. And if you just have to have that fettuccine alfredo, then go for it. Just eat half the portion, or maybe just a third, and you may have to do a few more laps around the block…but exercise, or lack there of, is another issue we will tackle later!

4

Beverage Choices

What is the best beverage to drink when you are trying to manage your weight? That's right, water, water, and more water. Yep, the old eight to ten glasses of water a day sermon. When counseling my clients on weight loss, this is one of the simplest concepts to present, yet one of the most resisted. I have had numerous individuals tell me that they just simply can't drink water. Period. And they won't give up their soda. And my answer is always a firm, "Then I guess you're not really serious about losing weight right now, are you?" You **can** drink water, and you **must**. Water is essential to hydrate your body and to promote proper metabolism of the food you eat. I have had clients tell me that they hate the taste of water. My response to that is simple: Learn to like it. People have gotten so used to quenching their thirsts with super-sized cola beverages that they have lost their taste for water! Heaven forbid they drink anything unflavored!

Numerous legitimate studies have been done on both diet and regular soda beverages that indicate that they are detrimental to our health. But, unless you are a health care provider interested in reading those kinds of studies, you're generally not going to hear a lot of bad publicity about drinking sodas. In fact, quite the opposite is true. The soft drink industry is a multi-billion dollar industry with powerful lobbyists. They have even managed to get their soda machines into our schools by giving kickbacks to those schools that allow them to bring in their vending machines. And television and magazines are inundated with beautiful young models quenching their thirst with their favorite sodas. They don't show those same models a few years later at the dental office getting their teeth capped or having huge cavities filled from years of having sugary, high acidic, carbonated beverages coat their teeth. (My husband is a dentist who has seen first hand the damage soda abuse can cause!) The soda industry's advertising tactics are just as shameful as cigarette advertisements.

Dental caries is just one ill effect of chronic soda abuse. Weight gain is the other. Recent studies have suggested that our bodies do not recognize the calories consumed from beverages in the same manner that it recognizes calories from food. Let me give you an example of what I mean by this. If you drink a super-sized soda with a regular hamburger and fries, your total calorie intake will be approximately 1500 calories. The large soda contributes 500 calories to this meal. Did you eat less of the hamburger and leave some fries to make up for the 500 calories you were getting from the soda? Probably not. Your body does not recognize that it should be getting full from the calories contributed by the soda, so you eat the same amount of food as you would if you were having a glass of water. And you are up an extra 500 calories for the day. Let's continue and I will show you how that 500 calories a day in soda can make a huge difference in your ability to lose weight on a weekly basis.

In order to understand how dramatically this affects your weight loss goals, you need to know that one pound equals 3500 calories. Therefore, you must decrease your caloric intake by 3500 calories to lose one pound in a week. You can choose to decrease your calories or increase your exercise to burn off more calories, or do a combination of the two. If you are drinking one super-sized soda a day, that is equals to, at least, 500 calories a day from soda. 500 calories times 7 days of the week equals 3500 calories for the week. Remember that 3500 calories equal one pound. Therefore, that is one pound of weight you could lose a week just by cutting out the soda you drink! "Ah!" you say, "I'll just substitute diet soda for the regular and cut out all the calories!" Well, that might help a bit, but some recent studies have shown that people who consume diet beverages aren't much better off in the weight loss game than their regular soda-drinking friends. Why? Well, the jury is still out on that one. The studies are not conclusive and researchers aren't quite sure why they are seeing that phenomenon. It may be simply that soda drinkers in general just aren't eating the healthiest of diets. Some other studies point to the fact that we may indeed be metabolizing some of those sugar substitutes as calories. But, whatever the facts may be, it is enough information to sell me on water as the beverage of choice to ensure successful weight management. And just like my advice with fast foods, soft drink beverages simply need to be eliminated from your diet. Please keep in mind that if you are a caffeinated cola junkie, you will need to decrease your cola intake gradually to prevent the severe headaches that can accompany caffeine withdrawal. The rest of you can decide whether going cold turkey on the sodas or gradually weaning yourself from them works best for you. Keep in mind, there is no one perfect way to change dietary habits; the important thing is to make the change.

Moving on to other beverage choices. Yes, there are a few other choices other than your daily water intake! I always recommend that my clients eat their nutrients versus drink them. However, some nutrients are just more conveniently available, or less caloric, in beverage form than in food form. An example of this is calcium. We have already touched on the importance of an adequate daily calcium intake in the prevention of osteoporosis. Unfortunately, calcium is one of the first nutrients to go when women diet, as they typically cut out milk and fatty dairy foods before anything else. And they generally will substitute diet beverages for their milk intake. But we won't beat that dead horse again! In general, women need approximately 1200 mg of calcium daily (men need about 1000 mg) to help prevent osteoporosis, a debilitating bone disease. Four-eight ounce glasses of milk provides this needed calcium. However, when managing your weight, it is not always possible to include four glasses of milk a day and stay within your calorie needs. If you are a small, middle-aged women who only needs 1200 to 1500 calories a day, (it's tough to be short), then it might be really hard to stay within your daily calorie needs with four glasses of milk contributing 360 calories. I am calculating skim milk calories here. 2% milk would contribute 480 calories. That is about 30 to 40 percent of your daily calorie intake in milk! And I won't even calculate whole milk, because that is just a dietary no-no. In fact, I recommend skim milk **only** to all of my clients. Just like the water thing, you can get used to it and it does taste good. It is simply a matter of retraining your taste buds over time. Trust me, if my husband can make the change from 2% to skim milk, you can, too. Although, he also eats tofu now, but that's another book!

Here is the plan when including milk in your daily calorie allotment: One, drink skim milk and skim milk only! Two, remember that you can meet your daily calcium requirements by including other good calcium choices, such as cheese, yogurt, and other low fat dairy products so you don't always need four cups of milk a day. Just watch your portion sizes and choose lower fat options because many dairy products are typically high fat foods. It is important to consider your nutrient needs when choosing a beverage. Our bodies can only absorb about 250-300 mg of calcium at a time. One eight-ounce glass of milk has about 250 mg of calcium in it. Therefore, one cup of milk is all you would need to fulfill your calcium needs at any one time, and any additional milk would basically be "empty calories" with no additional nutrient benefits.

The message here, is to measure out your eight-ounce glass of milk; and any additional beverage should be calorie-free, that is, water! That way you are not consuming any unnecessary calories with no nutritional gain. Just one last thought on the importance of meeting your daily calcium needs: Recent studies have indicated that dieters who maintain adequate calcium intake have more successful weight loss than those who fall short in meeting their daily calcium needs.

Research still continues on this subject, but scientists believe that calcium may play a vital role in fat metabolism.

Another daily vitamin need that can be met through beverage intake is vitamin C. One six-ounce glass of orange juice provides all the vitamin C you need for the day. Vitamin C is a water-soluble vitamin, which means consuming more than your body needs just gets flushed down the toilet, so to speak. Juices are generally calorically dense, so typically it is best to just eat a citrus fruit to get your daily vitamin C dose. Eating the whole fruit provides a little more satiety and nutrients from the fiber content. However, if you are going to drink juice, do so only to get your daily vitamin C dose in six ounces and again, any additional liquids should be non-caloric, that is, water! Are you getting the point?

It would be remiss to ignore one very caloric category of beverages—alcohol. This group includes beer, wine, all hard liquor, dessert liquors, and mixed drinks. Most often the dessert alcoholic beverages and mixed drinks will be the most caloric of the group, because of the added sugar from mixers or fat from creams. Alcohol can be a real calorie buster if not paid attention to. You can be diligent in your daily meal plan all week, but if you blow it with five beers in a weekend or two glasses of wine every night after work, you will be really packing in some extra calories. Alcoholic beverages lower your inhibitions, which can lead to over-indulging at the dinner table. So, although I believe in the beauty of an occasional glass of wine with dinner, a tasty beer with your pizza, or a margarita on the beach, just be careful not to over-indulge and add to the bulge.

Finally, regarding coffee and tea, these are calorie-free beverages. There is no harm in a cup or two of coffee or tea on a daily basis. In fact, many studies indicate that coffee, and especially tea, may provide beneficial antioxidants. When I say coffee, this does not include coffee drinks like cappuccinos or lattes or mochas at your local coffeehouse. These typical coffee drinks can be loaded with extra sugar and cream. Some of these beverages can contain 500 to 700 calories in a single small serving. And, be aware that, as with all caffeinated beverages, coffee and tea can act as a diuretic and increase your need for, guess what? Water!

5

Planning Daily Meals

How you spread your calories out throughout the day has a **huge** impact on your ability to control your daily food intake, and ultimately your weight. One of the first questions I ask a client is, "What and when do you eat during a typical day?" Probably the greatest dieting pitfall is skipping breakfast. And similar to the water lecture, this is a very simple concept, but again highly resisted. Eating breakfast is **the** single most important factor in maintaining portion control and stabilizing blood sugar levels and hormone levels to prevent daily food cravings and binge eating. Nine out of ten overweight people will skip breakfast or consume inadequate calories and/or protein in their morning meal. They argue that if they eat breakfast, it makes them nauseous or it makes them overeat for the rest of the day. To that, I say "fat chance." They have breakfast issues that must be dealt with! They may perceive that it makes them nauseous or tend to overeat, but the reality is that eating breakfast does neither. In fact eating a well-balanced breakfast can actually improve your metabolic rate (calorie burn) by as much as ten percent for the entire day. Furthermore, eating breakfast is the only way you will have successful, healthy weight loss and continued success with weight control.

Imagine the following situation: You ate dinner at 6:00 p.m. and a small evening snack at 8:00 p.m. and you went to bed. Your alarm goes off at 6:00 a.m. and you promptly get up for work. (Not too realistic, but stay with me here!) You skip breakfast and head out the door. You get to the office at 8:00 a.m., and you grab a cup of coffee on the way to your cubicle. It has now been approximately twelve hours since you've last eaten. Your body is essentially in a fasting state. Your blood sugar has bottomed out. The human body is very good at adapting and conserving calories when calorie deficiencies occur. It goes way back to survival of the fittest and making do with less food during the cold winter months when food supplies were limited and hunting was poor. Energy is conserved; that is, fewer calories are used, when food sources are limited. This can be likened to a bear conserving its energy during hibernation. So when you throw your body into a "false" period of starvation by skipping breakfast, not only are you setting yourself up for overeating and food cravings for the rest of the day, but you are also lowering your metabolic rate. Your body tries to conserve energy. Although you may be moving around, busily beginning your day, you are actually burning fewer calories than if you would have had a solid, healthy breakfast.

Now, to address the idea of a morning meal making you nauseous, I understand that not everyone is a morning person. But if your work schedule is such that you have to be at the office by 8:00 a.m., then you need to adjust your morning routine to work in breakfast at some point in the morning. Breakfast doesn't have to be the first thing on your agenda in the morning, and it doesn't have to be a full course ham and egg meal. The key, though, is to eat something, and that something should be a combination of a complex carbohydrate with a protein source to give your blood sugar both an immediate lift (from the carbohydrate) and some staying power (from the protein source and the fiber in the complex carbohydrate). A small amount of fat in the morning is also important to add some satiety to your meal.

Some examples of simple breakfast combinations are as follows:

- One cup of low fat yogurt mixed with a banana and ¼ cup whole grain cereal

- Whole-wheat toast with 1-2 tablespoons of peanut butter and 8-ounce skim milk

- ¾ cup of whole grain cereal with fruit and 8-ounce skim milk

- 1 hard-boiled egg, a slice of whole-wheat toast, and 6-ounce juice

- A grilled cheese sandwich (prepared with 1-ounce of cheese and no butter) and 6-ounce juice

These are just a few suggestions. I could list more, but you get the idea. An example of an unhealthy breakfast would be a donut or a pastry and a cup of coffee. Why? First, because a donut or pastry is laden with fat calories, which you simply don't need. And secondly, because, other than the fat, all you are giving your body as fuel is simple sugar. This goes right into your bloodstream, sends your blood sugar soaring, and then an hour (or less) later your blood sugar will come crashing down and you will likely experience a food craving. And what are you going to crave? That's right, something sweet or salty. Your body will crave a simple sugar. Why? Because, as I mentioned before, our natural instincts kick in when our blood sugar plummets an hour after eating that donut and our body is screaming, "Uh oh, I have to get my blood sugar back up to a normal level."

Consuming simple sugars is the quickest way to do that. Those sugars are found in convenience foods like cakes, cookies, pastries, candy bars, chips, or many people's favorite standby, soda.

One of my favorite excuses for not including breakfast is the famous; "I just don't have time in the morning!" My response? If it is important to you, you will find the time. If you have kids to get off to school in the morning, get them organized the night before. Make their lunches the night before, or better yet, have them get themselves organized for school and make their own lunches. Set your alarm fifteen minutes earlier and get up. You can find the time, and you can fit in breakfast…**if** it is a priority. Once again, this all comes back to what you as an individual want to do to eat healthy and feel good.

Once you have learned how to include a healthy breakfast into your daily routine, you will need to reevaluate the rest of your meal and snack times. The smartest, healthiest way to maintain stable blood sugar levels and thereby control food binges and food cravings is to eat several small "meals" throughout the day. You should aim to eat about 200-300 calories every two to three hours during the day. And the choices need to be appropriate. This eating pattern will vary with each individual depending on your work or play schedule for the day. It does require some thought and planning to have healthy food choices on hand. Each "mini meal" should consist of a protein and a complex carbohydrate. Some examples include: yogurt, cheese and crackers, a half of a peanut butter sandwich on whole wheat bread, or a piece of fruit and a handful of nuts. Again, the list could go on and on. Notice I didn't include a bag of potato chips or a candy bar from the vending machine!

Many families typically have a small breakfast, a larger lunch, and then a big dinner after work. This pattern is opposite from how your calories should be spread out during the day. It is healthier to consume the majority of your calories early in the day when you need those calories for daily tasks of living. Your evening meal should be the lightest meal of the day. A meat, potato, and vegetable meal, is not necessary every night, even for the kids. If you provide healthy food choices for their breakfast and lunch meals, they do not need a "balanced" evening meal. Sometimes my kids have a bowl of lightly buttered noodles and a glass of milk for dinner. I'm not at all concerned that they are lacking in their nutrient intake. I know that over the week's time they will be getting a varied diet and that variety will provide them with all the essential vitamins and minerals their growing bodies need. On busy days when I don't have time to cook, my family will enjoy a mixed green salad with cheese and crackers as our evening meal. These are the nights when we might enjoy a bowl of ice cream after dinner.

We are not uncomfortably stuffed from a large dinner, so dessert becomes part of our meal. Dessert is not a special "treat," it is just something we enjoy if we have had a light evening meal.

I do not want to assume that buttered noodles or a salad for dinner would work at your home. I only share these dinner options with you in order to get you to think outside of the box. So many of us have been programmed that mealtime, and especially dinnertime should be at a certain time each day, and should be a full course event, and that is simply not the case. If you focus on when you are truly hungry, and what nutrients your body needs, you will quit eating on an exact time clock with preconceived ideas of what foods should constitute a "meal."

6

Reshaping Your Food Life

I have had many clients tell me that they just can't get organized in the kitchen. Some of the excuses I have heard include: I'm too busy with work and the kids, or I hate to cook, or I hate to grocery shop. It is mind-boggling to me that some of the most organized people can't seem to get it together in the eating and food category! Ironically, the people who seem to have the most weight issues and food issues are those who spend very little time organizing or preparing their food and a lot of time obsessing over it! If your health and fitness are a priority, you will make organizing your daily food intake a priority. There is a big difference in making food a priority and making it an obsession. We all have to eat, and we all have to eat several times a day to be healthy. Therefore, it only makes sense to organize this part of your life and to give it some time and consideration so it doesn't become an obsession or just another chore. Too many people have simply forgotten the simple pleasure and joy of good food.

I'm not going to lie to you. Healthy eating takes a lot more time than eating junk. You have to grocery shop for the proper foods, organize your snacks and meals, and yeah, you may even have to wash some fruits and vegetables! It takes a bit more time than ripping open a bag of chips. On the other hand, once you get organized, it will become second nature and you will spend much less time than you think on food preparation. And, I guarantee you; in the long run it is a lot more satisfying, nutritionally and emotionally. For those of you who don't enjoy cooking, that's okay. You don't have to be a gourmet cook, but you still need to put some effort into grocery shopping and home food preparation. As I have discussed earlier, there is an array of really unhealthy convenience foods available, so too, there are just as many healthy convenience foods. You simply need to know what to look for, and you have to pay some attention to food labels. However, this does not have to be a science project. We will discuss grocery shopping and food labels in the next chapter, but for now, let's stick with organizational skills and food preparation. Food preparation can take minimal time at home and still be healthy. Once you have a well-stocked pantry of the essentials, your weekly grocery run will become much less time-consuming.

In order for you to get started on organizing your food life, you first need to organize your pantry and refrigerator and freezer. By simply keeping some basic supplies on hand, you can whip up an easy meal in no time, without resorting to fast food meals or high calorie processed foods. In chapter 7, I have provided a partial list of healthy, helpful food brand choices. Some of these brands make dinner helpers such as meatless chili, taco filling, sloppy joe sandwiches, or noodle dishes that are great pantry items to keep on hand when food preparation time is limited. Please keep in mind, that although all of our lives are busy, our meal preparation and our meal sit down time should be a part of our daily lives. It is not about how fast you can get food on the table, and then how fast can you eat it so that you can move on to other "things" you need to do. Time should be taken in the organization, preparation, presentation, and enjoyment of the meal. This doesn't have to mean a five-course meal every night. But stop to enjoy the entire food process. You have to eat! Make it fun and include other members of the family in the entire process. If you change your perception of mealtime, and look at it not as a chore but as an "event," it puts it in a whole different perspective. Any number of things you have to do in the course of a day can be looked at as a "chore," but if you change your outlook, you can change the outcome. What once was viewed as just another chore, can instead be an enjoyable daily event that you can look forward to. It is all a matter of perspective. Are there some days when you just can't sit and relax over a meal as long as other days? Of course, but that should be the exception, not the rule.

I have listed what I believe to be some of the essentials you should have on hand to make a simple healthy meal at home, in as timely a manner as possible. Your selection of spices and other staples will vary depending on your ethnic background and your cooking skills. This is simply a partial list to get you started. Again, refer to chapter 7 for helpful healthy brand names.

Pantry Essentials

Whole-wheat noodles

Taco shells

Whole grain rice

Pasta sauce

Low fat refried beans

Canned fruits

Canned beans (any variety)

Salad dressing

Whole grain cereal

Canned tuna

Refrigerator Essentials

Lettuce

Seasonal fruits (at least 1 variety)

Milk

Yogurt

High quality cheeses

Eggs or egg substitute

Skim milk

Freezer Essentials

Lean meat (any kind)

Skinless chicken breasts

Frozen fish

Veggie burgers

Whole wheat bread and buns

Frozen fruit (any variety)

Frozen vegetables (any variety)

Frozen yogurt or sherbet

With these basic food staples on hand, you can make just about any quick and easy meal or snack. A bag of frozen fruit and some low-fat yogurt allows you to blend up a nutritious, delicious fruit smoothie for an afternoon snack. Frozen veggie burgers or pre-making your own hamburger patties and freezing them, makes for a quick dinner. Always having the "fruit of the week" on hand lends to a great snack or a healthy compliment to a meal.

Let me give you an example of a simple, yet nutritious and delicious meal that you can prepare with the basic kitchen staples I have suggested from the previous list. Pasta: everyone's favorite and a quick and easy meal to prepare. There are just a couple of things to keep in mind with a pasta meal. One, buy whole-wheat pasta, and two, limit your portion size. Generally, whole-wheat pasta will taste pretty much the same as its white counterpart; however, the extra fiber will provide extra satiety and other nutritional benefits to your diet. You may find the texture more firm than white pasta, but that is a good thing as it allows you to chew your food and eat more slowly, both of which are important in the whole scheme of enjoying every bite that you put into your mouth. Eating should never be about how fast you can get the meal down, but instead, how much you are enjoying the taste of the food, and how nutritious it is.

On to the preparation part of the meal: you simply boil some water and cook the pasta. Open a jar of pasta sauce (most are low fat if you avoid the ones with the added meat) and heat the sauce up. Cut a slice of whole wheat French bread that you have taken from your freezer. You really need no butter on your bread because you will probably dip it in your sauce. Add a tossed salad…again from a bag if you want to save some effort in the kitchen, and a small amount of salad dressing. Remember, you are eating salad, not dressing…taste the green stuff, it's actually quite good when it's not all covered up with dressing. Slice an orange to go with your meal and presto! You have a meal that took less than thirty minutes to prepare, cost almost nothing, and is healthy and nutritionally balanced.

I can hear some of you screaming, "But wait, there is no meat in that meal! I can't do that!" Yes, you can. You do not have to be a tofu eating soy-aholic convert to eat healthy, but a few meatless meals won't kill you, and these meatless meals will help to limit the fat and calories in your overall meal plan. There are so many examples of simple healthy meals like this that you can prepare at home.

For those of you who still don't believe that you have time in your day to dedicate to food preparation, I say, make the time. The time is there, but you may have to first sit down and organize your day and your week to see what other obligations can be eliminated or delegated to free up some time for food organization and preparation. I suggest this challenge: For a two week period take some time away from one of your other daily activities, say for example watching television or emailing friends. Take an inventory of your pantry and refrigerator and freezer. Get a notebook and write down a simple menu for the week and list the groceries you would need to make those meals. Go to the grocery store and buy just those items, completely skipping the cookie and chip and soda aisles. Be careful not to be too zealous in the fruit and vegetable department. My advice to clients who are trying to increase their daily fruit and vegetable intake is to take it slowly. If you go from eating no fresh fruits and vegetables to trying to meet the five a day requirement, you are in for some major gastrointestinal upset. Not to mention the money you will waste by having to throw out all the stuff that rots while you are recovering from the bloat! I generally suggest that when you are first getting the hang of a weekly menu and grocery list, that you only buy two vegetables…unless your meals include some veggie stir fries. And limit your fruit choices to one or two varieties. For example, if you know you like a banana every morning on your cereal, buy a bunch of bananas for the week. Then, buy one other variety of fruit of your choice that is in season and on sale that particular week. For example, in the winter, when oranges are in season and on sale, I will buy one bag of oranges for the family for the week. If grapefruit are on sale the next week, I buy a bag of them. This way, you finish what you buy without it spoiling before you can eat it all. You aren't overwhelmed by too much variety at home, which means you don't have to think or make a conscious decision about which fruit to eat. If you have oranges that week, you eat oranges, simple. And, you still are able to include a variety of fruits and vegetables in your overall diet.

When you hear health professionals advocating eating a variety of foods in your diet, they don't necessarily mean that it has to be completely varied every day, just over a period of time. It's quite all right to eat oranges and bananas one week and apples and pears the next. You don't have to eat one apple, one pear, one orange, and one banana all in one day. That most definitely takes too much planning and mental thought to be doable on a daily basis. Most of us don't have a smorgasbord of different foods available to us every day. It gets frustrating to eat such a varied diet daily, and what people end up doing is just completely giving up and not eating any fruits or vegetables because it all becomes too overwhelming.

7

Grocery Shopping and the Skinny on Food Labels

I have already covered a little bit about grocery shopping in the previous chapter regarding buying perishables such as fruits and vegetables. But let me review a few other key topics when it comes to grocery shopping. I'm assuming that most people have a budgeted amount of money to spend weekly on groceries. You **can** shop healthfully and economically. In fact, dollar for dollar, you will spend more money if you are purchasing unhealthy food choices. Prepackaged cookies, chips, crackers, bakery items and other convenience foods cost a lot of money. How do you think they pay for all of their marketing and advertising?

The other day in the grocery store I heard a young mother tell her little girl that she couldn't have the grapes this week because they weren't on sale and were too expensive. Well, I couldn't help myself, I peeked into her cart, and what do you think I saw? I saw a name brand package of chocolate donuts (I'm assuming they were on sale), sugar-coated cereal, and a bag of chocolate sandwich cookies (the expensive ones, you know which ones I'm talking about!) and a case of soda (you already know how I feel about that!) I bit a hole in my tongue and walked on. I really wanted to confront that mother's food issues right there on the spot and I almost screamed, "Are you kidding! Grapes are too expensive, but you have all that other junk in your cart!" Now granted, I've told my own kids to pick the fruit or the veggie of the week instead of the more expensive out-of-season choice, but I also don't have a cart full of expensive junk food to boot. You can save yourself a lot of money and calories by simply skipping the chip and cookie and soda aisles, at least initially, until you have learned how to make appropriate choices from those aisles.

Let's discuss food labels. The interpretation of food labels is probably my least favorite nutritional topic. However, it is a necessary evil, and it would be neglectful from a professional standpoint to ignore the subject. Plus, you might as well know, I have math issues, and reading and understanding food labels involves a lot of math.

As a registered dietitian, I find food labels misleading, difficult to read, almost impossible to understand, and too confusing for most people to apply to their daily lives! I don't know how the average mere mortal is supposed to figure it all out! Every time I think I've got it down, they add a different category to the label. The newest is the PERCENT DAILY VALUE. Now, I know the daily value information has been around for a while and has the American Dietetic Association's seal of approval, but forgive me, I'm still getting used to the food pyramid versus the basic four food groups. To me, the "**BASIC 4**" says it all. This is a very simple concept. This I can grasp. Why confuse the issue when we already have enough issues! I am not a big fan of getting all caught up in how many grams of this or that you should have a day. When you are just beginning to learn about healthy eating, it can be helpful to know **about** how many calories are in some basic foods and beverages and **about** how many calories you will need per day to maintain or reach a certain weight goal. However, overall, I think it is much more constructive to learn how to make appropriate food choices and control portion sizes than to calculate exact calorie, fat, protein, or carbohydrate values.

Although I would much prefer to avoid the subject altogether, let's review the basics of nutritional label reading 101. Maybe I can simplify and demystify the whole subject for all of us, by sharing just a few common sense guidelines. First of all, if you are like most people, you don't have the time or the desire to spend ten minutes reading the contents of each box or package you take off your grocer's shelf. There have been times when I am embarrassed to say I have spent ten minutes looking at a label and **still** not figured out whether it is a healthy choice or not! Kind of like when you are trying to compare prices of a five-pound bag of flour with a ten-pound bag of flour. If the unit price isn't printed on the shelf, I'm not doing the math! Talk about basic math issues!

Let's start with the NUTRITION FACTS part of the food label. In this section, you will be given the serving size and the amount of calories, fat, protein, carbohydrates and most often fiber content. I will use the example of a package of six cheese-filled crackers. The serving size is one whole package (six crackers). The calories for the entire package are 200 and the fat calories are 100. Now, even if you have a few math issues like me, you can see that 50 percent of the calories from these crackers are attributed to fat calories. When trying to determine if a food is too high in fat to include regularly in your diet, you can simplify the process by just dividing the total fat calories by the total calories of the food. If the fat content is greater than 30 percent, then this food should be limited in your diet.

The simplest way to put this is that no more than 30 percent of your daily total calories should come from fat. Therefore, most of the foods you eat should get less than 30 percent of their calories from fat. The goal is to limit your daily fat intake, **not** to severely restrict it.

In the above example, I chose to use fat percentage because, in general, when you are trying to limit poor food choices, you are going to be trying to limit those foods that are highest in calories. Most of those foods are likewise the foods with the highest fat content. The rest of the nutritional labeling may be completely irrelevant to your needs.

Earlier in this chapter I mentioned the PERCENT DAILY VALUE information provided on food labels. There have been many debates on whether providing the percent daily value information is helpful or not to most people. You can probably guess my feelings on that issue. I personally think that the percent daily value information is erroneous and terribly confusing. The label will tell you that percent daily values are based on a 2,000-calorie diet. Some labels will even tell you that your daily values may be higher or lower, depending on your calorie needs. Well, duh! They are saying that the "majority" of people need 2,000 calories a day. That little claim makes the information even that much more confusing. As I said in the beginning of this book, we are all individuals; no one diet works for everyone, and no exact number of calories per day works for everyone. Each of us has our own individual calorie needs depending on our gender, body type, age, and activity level. It is crazy to pick out a calorie number and assign it to the general population to use as a dietary guideline. I will use myself as an example here. I am "on the verge" of 40 years old, and barely 5 feet 2 inches tall. I exercise daily. Despite my regular exercise habits, I could never eat 2,000 calories every day and maintain a healthy weight! Taking my age and height into consideration, it would be a slow steady weight gain for me on that many calories every day. And it is unrealistic to assume that someone eats the same exact number of calories every day. Some days I may eat more or less than that one specific number. Therefore, in my opinion you can completely ignore the percent daily value information provided on food labels.

Now that we have the percent daily value part of the label simplified, let's look at the information listed under CONTENTS. There are two ingredients that I believe are the most important to avoid if you are trying to follow a healthy diet. One is high fructose corn syrup and the other is partially hydrogenated fat. High fructose corn syrup is just a fancy name for sugar, sugar, and more sugar. Most often you will find this ingredient in juices, cereals, and other high sugar processed foods. Partially hydrogenated fat is a fancy name for "really unhealthy fat source." You will find partially hydrogenated fat in most chips, snack foods, crackers, cereals, and baking mixes. If the ingredients listed include partially hydrogenated soybean, cottonseed oil and/or canola oils, put the product back on the shelf. You don't want to purchase it. Simply put, this is the worst type of fat a product can contain. One thing to note when looking at the list of ingredients in the CONTENTS section is that ingredients are always listed in the order of highest concentration to lowest concentration. Therefore, if high fructose corn syrup or partially hydrogenated fat is listed as the first, second, or third ingredient, that product will have a very high amount of that ingredient in it and it is most certainly a poor food choice.

Let me take a moment to clarify why hydrogenated fat is such a poor nutritional choice. Hydrogenation involves altering the chemical bond of the fat molecule, which some scientific studies have indicated may increase your LDL levels of cholesterol (the bad cholesterol) and may increase your risks of some cancers. Again, you will find that hydrogenated fat is in almost all prepackaged convenience foods, including, but not limited to, convenience dinner helpers, snack crackers, chips, cakes and cookies, packaged breads, pastries and bagels. It is in most butter substitutes, although there are now a few good butter alternatives that actually advertise "no hydrogenated fats" on their labels for that small percentage of the consumer population that is starting to figure out the game!

Just by eliminating most, or at best, all of the foods that contain high fructose corn syrup and hydrogenated fat, you will begin to eliminate those "junk" foods that are just adding all those extra calories and fat to your basic diet. If you make that one change in your food purchasing habits, you would be amazed at all the junk you can cut out of your diet, and how much healthier your choices would be without even making any other changes. If you check the labels and omit the foods that contain high fructose corn syrup and hydrogenated fats, you may initially become frustrated and feel like you just don't have any other choices. Well, that is simply not true. If you do a little exploring and check the labels on alternative sources, you will see that there are many, many other more healthful choices. But, this is where you have to do some work. Most major food chains now have at least one aisle dedicated to "healthy" choices or will place those choices right next to the bad guys.

Some of you may have to get over your preconceived ideas that all things labeled "organic" and or "healthy" are more expensive and less tasty. That is just not true. Maybe ten years ago I would have agreed with that statement, but today there are so many great choices available. You just have to be willing to try a few of them and yes, your taste buds may need to adjust a bit. You will learn to appreciate the taste of a real corn chip versus the plastic taste of the most popular brand. The following is a list of food brands that are healthy alternatives and do not contain high fructose corn syrup or hydrogenated fats. Please note that this list is not all-inclusive and that there are many other healthful choices available if you just take the time to do some basic investigating. Also, please note that just because these brands do not use high fructose corn syrup or hydrogenated fats does not automatically make them low calorie or low fat food choices. You still need to check basic fat content as discussed earlier and limit your portion sizes of all foods.

A partial list of "healthful" food brand choices as alternatives to more popular brands:

Guiltless Gourmet chips

Garden of Eaten' chips

Fantastic brand dinner helpers

Healthy Harvest pastas

Mi-Del brand crackers

Health Valley brand cookies and crackers

Terra brand potato chips

Cedarlane frozen foods

Boca frozen foods

Lightlife soy products

As I alluded to earlier, it is much more cost-effective to make healthy choices versus the foods that are just plain junk. Will you pay more on occasion for some of the healthier choices? Yes, maybe. But, what most people fail to take into consideration is the long-term medication and health care costs of living an unhealthy life of poor nutrition that leads to obesity, heart disease, cancer, and diabetes. And that doesn't even take into consideration the value you put on your quality of life. Quality of life suffers tremendously when you live with one or more of these nutritionally related illnesses. So when you really think that bag of apples is too expensive compared to that bag of cookies...think again.

8

Hidden Calories and Diet Food Choices

Now in this next discussion of hidden calories, some of you may think that I am contradicting myself by suggesting that you should measure out some of the foods you eat. The key here is **some**. I am not talking about measuring and weighing and recording everything you take in on a daily basis. But, the cold hard truth is that some foods are so calorically dense, and so well hidden in your daily intake, that it is best to measure out the amount you are using to prevent overuse.

Many times it can seem as if you aren't really overeating, but the calories are there in what are called "hidden" calories. Hidden calories are those calories you get by adding condiments or flavorings to your foods. For example, that table-spoon or two of margarine or butter you melted into your vegetables while they were cooking. Or that quarter cup of olive oil you used just to keep the stir-fry from sticking to the pan. Whether you are using a healthy fat choice or not, calories like these add up and they can have a tremendous impact on your daily calorie intake. You need to be cautious when using these hidden fats. In fact, the best way to handle this issue is to simply eliminate as many hidden calorie sources as you can. You simply don't need to add any margarine or butter when cooking vegetables. Remember that you want to taste the vegetable, not the butter. If you want to taste butter, eat butter, but don't hide the real flavor of the foods you are preparing. When you are stir-frying or sautéing, use nonstick cookware and non-caloric cooking spray. If you have to add a little fat, use just a tablespoon of olive oil or canola oil. Measure it out, don't just pour in the oil to coat the bottom of the pan. You will most definitely use way too much. And although olive oil or other vegetable oils are healthier choices than butter or lard, the calories still add up and can sabotage your weight control efforts.

In addition to the hidden fat and calories used in cooking, there are other sources including salad dressings and butter or margarine used at the table. Salad dressings are by nature calorically dense, unless you are using diet varieties, which we will talk about next. The best way to handle salad dressings is to use a tablespoon to measure out your portion size on a salad. One or two tablespoons are all you need on an average sized salad. Some people find it helpful to serve the dressing in a separate bowl and dip their forks first into the dressing and then into the salad. This helps automatically portion out the amount you use. As for the butter or margarine on the table, simply don't even serve it. You just don't have to add any butter or margarine to anything once you are at the table. If you are having a slice of bread, a hot roll or a muffin with a meal, eat it plain. Taste the muffin, not the butter. You will cut down on a tremendous amount of fat calories in this way without really much effort and without counting a single calorie!

Other condiments that will add up to a lot of calories in a hurry include sour cream, gravy, dips, and any other cream type sauces. Again, the easiest way to control these calorie sources is simply to eliminate them. Easy as can be! After awhile, you won't even miss those foods, and you will wonder why you ever bothered with them in the first place. Always remember, **taste the real food**. If the food is so bad that you have to mask it with sauces and butters, then it may not be worth eating in the first place. Either that or you may need to reevaluate your cooking skills!

And, don't forget those extra calories hidden in your coffee or tea. Again, it is a taste change issue. Learn to enjoy your coffee black and your tea without sugar. You will be amazed at how refreshing both beverages can be when you drink them unsullied. All tastes are learned tastes.

Next, I would like to discuss the issue of diet foods. Ugh. Even the sound of "diet" foods sounds bad! Now please, don't misunderstand me here. There are some good low fat or reduced fat food choices available that you should be purchasing instead of their higher fat counterparts. All of the low fat or no fat dairy products are smart choices. These include skim milk, low fat cottage cheese, skim milk cheeses, and low fat yogurts. Low fat or fat free cream cheese and sour cream can be substituted for their higher fat versions in most recipes.

There are also some good non-hydrogenated fat substitutes that can be used for baking. Many of these are made from apple puree. Just look in the baking section of the grocery store. Other than the low fat dairy alternatives previously mentioned, it is my opinion that most of the other "diet" or low fat food choices may simply sabotage your weight management goals and your healthy eating goals. I will need to explain the role of insulin and weight gain to help you understand this concept.

Insulin is a hormone that is released by the pancreas whenever carbohydrates are eaten, and in smaller amounts when protein is eaten. Insulin's job is to stimulate cells to open up and allow the glucose (the sugar in carbohydrates) to enter the cells and be used for energy. Simply put, when we eat carbohydrates, our blood glucose rises and our insulin rises. That increase in insulin tells the body **not** to burn fat and to move any extra fat in the blood into storage. What does this have to do with low-fat diets? When fat is removed from a high fat food, sugar is added to replace the fat. A good example of this is regular peanut butter versus low fat peanut butter. If you compare the labels, 2 tablespoons of regular peanut butter and 2 tablespoons of low fat peanut butter have the same amount of calories, approximately 200 calories. How can that be if one is less fat? Simple. They haven't just omitted the fat calories but instead the fat calories have been replaced with sugar calories. When you apply this concept to low fat diets, you can see that when the fat in your diet decreases, the carbohydrate in your diet generally will increase, thus raising your glucose level and therefore your insulin level. These high levels of insulin discourage fat burning, cause blood sugar lows as the extra insulin works to empty the blood of extra glucose, and set you up for sugar cravings. This concept is what has fueled all the hype on carbohydrates being "bad" and it has contributed to the high protein/high fat diet fads.

Moving on to the butter versus margarine debate. I am a firm believer in using "real" butter when preparing "real" foods. Now that is not to say I don't use the previously mentioned fat substitutes in some recipes. In general, it has been my experience that if a recipe for a baked product calls for butter, you can substitute half the amount of butter with a non-hydrogenated fat substitute. Again, the use of real butter comes down to taste and portion control. The taste of real butter goes a long way. If you use a small amount in whatever you are preparing it can greatly enhance the taste and flavor of a recipe. I also believe that the amount of saturated fat that you will get from real butter is a much healthier choice than the hydrogenated or trans fats found in margarines and most butter substitutes.

Often times I will have a new client confess that they have tried just about every diet out there, and that they have serious doubts that anything I have to tell them is going to be any more successful than what they have already tried. My first question is, "Do most of the diets you've tried restrict fat?" They always look at me incredulously and answer, "Well of course. Isn't dieting all about having the willpower to follow a low-fat diet?" The answer to that is a firm no. Being prudent with the amount of daily fat you consume, and severely restricting it, are two completely different concepts. What most people need to understand is that they have trouble staying on a low fat diet, not because they lack willpower, but in fact, because an adequate amount of fat in the diet is necessary to add satiety to their meal plan, stabilize their blood sugar levels, and prevent food cravings.

The guideline I personally use when deciding whether to use a low fat food choice or its higher fat counterpart, is simply taste and nutritional value. (You may have a little work to do regarding redefining what tastes good to you.) I firmly believe that everything you put in your mouth should taste good and should also play a part in your nutritional well being. And your nutritional well being includes satisfying your emotional needs for food as well as your physiological needs. Let me give you a couple of examples of how I make low fat versus regular fat food choices for myself. Example one: I choose to use skim milk because I drink milk for the nutritional benefits it provides in its calcium and protein content. I choose skim milk versus 2% or whole because it saves me a tremendous amount of calories and I would rather save those calories for something else in my daily meal plan. Example two: I use real butter on my air-popped popcorn. I measure out two tablespoons of butter for one half cup of unpopped popcorn. The amount of butter I am using is not unreasonable. I thoroughly enjoy the taste of real butter on my popcorn, and the fat it provides is necessary to help keep my blood sugar levels stable and provide a level of satiety in my daily meal plan. Those are the "unconsciously" conscious decisions that you should think about as you make food choices throughout the day. When you take time to recognize and acknowledge what causes you to make certain food choices, you will be on your way to controlling and monitoring what and why you eat based on nutritional and healthy living ideals. You will begin to enjoy organizing your daily food intake instead of obsessing over your daily food intake.

In the next chapter, I will discuss just what I mean by satisfying "emotional" nutritional needs.

9

Emotional Eating Issues

Until this point, I have been focusing mostly on how to make appropriate food choices using healthy nutritional guidelines. But the truth is that most of us don't make daily food choices simply because of the nutritional value of a particular food. We eat to nourish our bodies, but we also eat to fulfill emotional needs. I am not saying that eating for emotional reasons is right or wrong, only that it is. Emotional eating is virtually unavoidable. We all do it. Who doesn't have memories that trigger certain undeniable cravings for a particular food? For example, the smell of a turkey roasting on Thanksgiving or the aroma of freshly baked chocolate chip cookies hot out of the oven. Other than the topic of exercise resistance, emotional eating is one of the most difficult areas to tackle.

Food is so personal, and the rituals, traditions, and experiences that surround each individual's food habits can be so ingrained that often as a clinician, I find myself treading lightly when first addressing this topic. An "attack" on an individual's deeply rooted food habits and rituals can be misconstrued as an "attack" on that individual's self-image. However, to gain control over unhealthy food habits or to discover why you may have a particular craving at a particular time, it is mandatory to delve into the past and uncover what may be triggering certain consistent patterns of emotional eating.

Many of us in the baby boom generation grew up in households where waste, and in particular, food waste was an absolute no-no. Our parents lived through the Great Depression and the "clean your plate" mentality was necessary because you might not have a plate to clean the next day! When such messages are drilled into a child's head meal after meal, day after day, those are hard lessons to unlearn. It can take years to let go of the guilt associated with not "cleaning your plate."

I am not advocating that we waste food, only that we recognize that smaller portions or leftovers are always viable options for anyone, especially a child. I have seen families who serve their kids huge portions and then tell them that they

31

cannot have dessert unless they finish their entire meal. These are confusing messages to a child. One, a child may never discover what I refer to with my own children as their personal "shut off valve." That is, they will not be able to make the physical and mental connection between being comfortably full, because they are expected to finish their meal whether they are full or not. Secondly, by holding back dessert as a "reward" for finishing their meal, they may feel as if they have to eat dessert whether they are hungry for it or not. Dessert must be special if they are only allowed to have it if they have cleaned their plate! So you can see how these early food messages can play a huge role in your eating behaviors and emotional eating later in life. As unintentional as these food messages may be, a child can misconstrue the messages. A child's interpretation often becomes, "You're a good kid if you "clean your plate" and you can have a "treat," that is, dessert, if you do!" Two wrong messages!

Please keep in mind that not all food memories have to be bad memories to trigger emotional eating. Holiday eating is a good example of this. Thanksgiving is a holiday in most families that is associated with many delicious comfort foods and feasting all day long until you burst! As a child, I just accepted that this was what the holiday was all about, and that you were supposed to eat until you popped! It took years of retraining my emotional food memories to realize I could enjoy the day, the festivities, and most of all the food, in a healthy way, without feeling like a bloated pig by the end of the day. My mom is an exceptionally good cook, so it was really hard to not stuff yourself on her once a year specialties! And guess what I discovered? They sell turkey at the grocery store all through the year, so you can have turkey and all the fixings any time you want! You don't have to gorge yourself all in one day because you won't get it again until next year! My mom even started to cook turkey and all the trimmings in July, just because she could!

This seems like a good place to reflect on one major food issue I have regarding the subject of emotional eating. The use of the word "treat." I absolutely despise the word "treat" when associated with food. And it is a huge mistake I see parents and teachers make all the time. Food should **never,** and I mean **never** be used as a "reward" or "treat." And, on the same notion, food should never be withheld as a punishment. Food should not be used in either manner at any time under any circumstance. I have seen teachers give "treats" or "rewards" in the form of candy to students who get perfect marks on papers or for being "good" in class. It sends a wrong message to a child. It says, "Candy is good and desirable, and if I am good I get candy." Wrong message. Those messages can lead to deeply ingrained emotional food issues that are terribly hard to unlearn. If a reward is necessary for good work done, give the child a sticker, an eraser, or an extra privilege, but don't give food. There is no gray area in this situation. It just simply should not be done, ever. Period.

Kids are impressionable and they are always watching and learning from the examples we set. I have memories of my mom serving us kids just a small juice glass full of grapes. I always wanted more, but she always said no. I thought they were a "special treat" because we only got a small portion and never got seconds. It wasn't until years later when I asked my mom why she rationed grapes that I learned that it was because grapes were expensive, and with six kids to feed, she had to ration them out! I still think of grapes in the way that most people think of a decadent piece of chocolate! The moral of this story is that if something is restricted or limited you are going to want to overindulge in it just out of pure defiance!

At this point, I would like to challenge you to stop reading here. Take a few minutes to reflect on whatever "food" messages you were sent as a child. Did you take comfort in food because you didn't have an adult in your life that could provide you with emotional support and comfort? Were you offered "treats" for getting good grades, or for accomplishing a task, or for being "good"? Were you sent to bed without supper for being "bad"? Were you a shy child, who had a hard time making friends, so you turned to food as a friend? Take some time and reflect upon these questions. Write down any memories that you have that may trigger emotional eating for you as an adult. Once you identify these memories and how you reacted to them, they become so much easier to correct. If these memories are causing you to have unhealthy "emotional" food issues now, then it is time to reevaluate your responses to them and change your emotional eating behaviors. And remember, not all of your memories need to be bad memories to trigger overeating for emotional reasons. I had a loving family and a happy childhood, but even so I can reflect on both good and bad examples of food memories that trigger emotional eating in me to this very day. What matters now is how I choose to respond to those emotional food triggers, and how I make them work for me in choosing a healthy food life as an adult.

Once you have taken some time to reflect on what may be contributing to any problem emotional eating habits you may have, it is time to move on to some concrete tactics that you can use to change your eating behaviors. The following are a couple of ideas that might help you put a stop to emotional overeating:

If you have been programmed to clean your plate, then take a smaller plate or take smaller portions. Remember that excessive portion size is one of the biggest downfalls in weight management for most people. If you discover that you have taken too much and are full, stop eating! Put your fork down and take a breather. Don't just go into autopilot and finish the whole meal. Take time for your brain to register if you are truly full or not. Do whatever you have to do. If you can't bear to throw away any food, put it away as leftovers. Leftovers can be a great alternative to fast food lunches. If you can't stand the thought of leftovers, then give it to the dog. Just get rid of it.

If you have ever taken an economics class, you have probably learned about the law of diminishing returns. Simply put, this law purports that when you make a profit you generally will reach a peak, a point where you can go no further and your costs of making the product exceed that product's profitability. It is the old bell curve in action. The same thing happens when we eat. You reach a point of physical and psychological satiety where that next bite is just not quite as satisfying or thrilling as the first. As an example, imagine going to your favorite bakery and ordering a double fudge chocolate torte. You slice a generous piece, and sit down to truly enjoy every bite. The first bite is outrageous. The second bite just melts in your mouth and the chocolate literally explodes on your taste buds. (Am I killing you here?) You continue to eat your generous slice of cake, but as you eat it, you realize that with each bite your enjoyment of it is just a little bit less than the bite before. You are beginning to feel full and you can't quite taste all of the different chocolate flavors that you experienced in the first few bites. Your taste buds have become somewhat desensitized from the initial chocolate explosion. Each bite is beginning to taste just like the bite before it. This is the point of the law of diminishing returns. As you near the end of the piece of cake, each bite is not quite as luscious and delicious and satisfying as those first bites. That is the theory you should always keep in mind, especially if you are satisfying a craving. You don't have to eat the whole piece of cake or the entire bag of cookies. If you stop and pay attention to the law of diminishing returns, you may be satisfied with eating just half of the piece of cake or just one or two cookies instead of the entire bag. If you pay attention to this phenomenon, stopping when you are satisfied can become a natural response, and you will find yourself saying "no thank you" comfortably and sincerely much more often.

Every time you think about eating something, think about **why** you are eating it. Are you physiologically hungry? Is your stomach growling? Are you tired? Are you lonely or depressed? Are you bored? Are you happy and "celebrating" with friends? If you really stop to think about why you are eating, and focus on only eating when you are truly physiologically hungry, you will eliminate many, many mindless calories. If you are tired, don't eat; take a nap. If you are bored, don't eat; go for a walk or find something interesting to do. If you are sad or lonely, don't eat; call a friend instead. Just tuning into emotional eating, knowing that it is normal, and that you can control it, will give you the confidence and ability to change your emotional eating habits. The first step is to realize that emotional eating is real and that everyone struggles with this issue from time to time. The second step is to identify your own personal emotional food "issues." And the final step is to modify your behavior in response to those emotional cues.

Conquering the pitfalls of emotional eating will take time. You won't be successful each time, but you will gain insight into why, what, and how you eat for reasons other than real hunger. Controlling emotional eating habits can be empowering and enlightening. The first time you are successful in identifying your emotional needs and satisfying them appropriately and without food, you will be so excited and proud of yourself. It will be a huge light bulb moment in your life!

10

Issues with Fad Diets

There are so many fad diets, quick fixes, and magic pills on the market that I can't possibly cover the faults in all of them in one book. But, I can highlight some of the main problems with why they don't work. First of all, any diet or pill promising quick weight loss just won't work. Think of it logically. You didn't gain the extra weight overnight, so you aren't going to be able to lose it overnight either. As I mentioned earlier in the book, a safe and effective weight loss is one to two pounds per week. If you lose weight any faster than this, you will be losing water weight and lean body tissue (muscle). So the only way to lose weight permanently is to lose it slowly over a reasonable period of time. If you gained 20 pounds in one year, then it is a good chance that it will take you just that amount of time to lose that amount of weight. That is not said to discourage you in your efforts. It is simply realistic. It takes time to change food behaviors and to learn to change the lifestyle behaviors that contributed to your weight gain. Give yourself a break, and take the time to make a real commitment to lifestyle changes, and you will be successful in managing your weight.

In previous chapters, I have explained the reasons why low calorie and low fat diets do not work. Simply put, if you starve yourself, you lower your overall metabolic rate and in the end burn fewer calories, which sabotages your weight loss efforts. Plus, low calorie, low fat diets are difficult to stick to for any length of time, and most people will return to their old "bad" eating habits as soon as, or even before they have reached their weight goals. This is the classic yo-yo diet syndrome.

I mentioned the high protein, low carbohydrate diets in the chapter on hidden calories and diet foods. The most popular of these diets is the Atkins' Diet. High protein, low carbohydrate diets gained popularity when the role of insulin control and high carbohydrate intake was studied. Remember, a high carbohydrate intake causes more insulin to be released, which in turn causes fluctuations in a person's blood glucose levels, which ultimately contributes to food cravings and binge eating. Therefore, the premise of the high protein, low carbohydrate diet is to lower blood glucose levels, thereby lowering insulin levels and avoiding food cravings. The idea behind the diet is right on. However, the problem with most high protein, low carbohydrate diets, is that they promote the extreme. The amount of protein these diets want you to consume is too excessive and places undue stress on the kidneys. Following excessively high protein diets can cause permanent kidney damage. Also, diets high in protein are generally high in total and saturated fat. These diets promote eating a large amount of meat and dairy products, which are typically higher fat foods. High fat diets are associated with poor lipid profiles and coronary artery disease. What these diets fail to mention is that yes, lowering your carbohydrate intake is desirable, but you can lose weight simply by doing just that. If you cut out all the high calorie carbohydrate loaded junk foods like soda, candy bars, cookies, pies, pastries, and snack chips, you will lose weight without even changing your protein intake! In the end, these extremely high protein diets prove too difficult for people to follow for a long period of time, so again you have the issue of immediate weight loss without the benefit of learning how to make the safe long-term dietary changes necessary to continue with weight management.

Liquid diets don't work either. Why? Because, again, you can't stay on them forever, and they don't teach you how to improve your eating habits. When you go off the diets and return to your old eating habits, you will regain the weight. This holds true for diets that promote using their own foods and/or meal replacement bars instead of "real" foods. When you quit buying their "diet" foods and resume old eating habits, you will regain the weight. The only thing that will be thinner is your pocket book.

There are some prescription weight loss medications that may be helpful in the initial phases of weight loss. Most of these prescriptions work in two ways. They contain a drug that acts as an appetite suppressant and they contain a drug that is a metabolic stimulant. You may feel more hungry when you first start to change your eating habits because you will be reducing your calorie intake just by cutting out the "junk" we have talked about earlier. Therefore, the appetite suppressant can be helpful in taming your initial hunger pangs. However, as you adjust to a lower, healthier calorie intake, the suppressant will become less effective. And, keep in mind, as we have discussed earlier, we rarely eat purely for appetite reasons, so the medication does nothing to quell emotional eating. The metabolic stimulant can also be helpful in the initial phases of weight management. The stimulants work by boosting your metabolic rate (calorie burn), which can be helpful until you get a regular exercise routine in place. Again, the stimulant will become less effective over time. The use of weight loss medications should always be combined with nutritional counseling and regular medical checkups. They should only be prescribed to those people who are willing to make nutritional lifestyle changes, which will ensure their continued success with life long weight management. Prescription weight loss medications should never be used long-term, and should be discontinued if the patient does not participate actively in nutritional counseling sessions and an exercise program.

11

Nutritional Supplements

I am not a big fan of nutritional supplements. Let me give you my take on the whole issue. Long story short, I think most supplements are simply a waste of money. Nutritional and dietary supplements are a huge industry. Although improvements have been made within the industry, there is still a lack of standards and regulations that determine the exact quality of ingredients that make up certain supplements.

The number of supplemental choices available is overwhelming, to say the least. There are protein supplements, energy enhancing supplements, mood altering supplements, and vitamin and mineral supplements. The list goes on and on. Even as a nutritional expert, I find the choices mind boggling, confusing, and I don't mind admitting, just a little scary! You almost need to have a Ph.D. in biochemistry in order to know how to safely use most supplements.

If you have a medically diagnosed vitamin or mineral deficiency, supplementation to correct that deficiency may be medically prudent. For example, if you have been diagnosed with an iron deficiency anemia, iron supplementation as one mode of medical treatment, may be necessary. Or, if you have a condition such as osteoporosis, which is directly related to a dietary deficiency of calcium, oral supplementation may be warranted. Keep in mind, however, that while you are trying to correct a known deficiency through supplements, you should also be working on improving your nutritional habits to include foods that are rich in the deficient nutrient. Many studies have shown that our bodies absorb certain nutrients better when that nutrient is supplied through food, versus supplement form. There are certain food interactions that enhance the absorption of specific nutrients. For example, the protein, sugars, and vitamin D found in cow's milk enhance calcium absorption. Vitamin C enhances iron absorption. The interaction between various foods and the absorption of essential nutrients cannot be overlooked.

In the previous chapter on fad diets, I discussed the pitfalls of high protein diets, liquid supplements, and meal replacement bars. Unless you are a professional athlete or an Olympic hopeful, protein supplements are not necessary. So save your money and leave the protein supplements on the grocery shelf. As far as weight loss supplements, such as powdered drink mixes or meal replacement bars, they can be used **occasionally** in place of a meal, but remember, using liquid supplements, powder supplements, or energy bars as meal replacements doesn't teach you how to manage real foods in your everyday life.

A daily multivitamin is one supplement that may be nutritionally and economically prudent. None of us eats perfectly healthy every day of our lives. Therefore, a daily multivitamin can help safeguard you from possible nutrient deficiencies. But, I do want to clarify one misconception that many of my clients seem to have regarding multivitamins. I have had clients profess that multivitamin supplements give them an energy boost. A multivitamin does **not** give you an energy boost. Only calories from carbohydrates, protein, and fat can give you energy. A vitamin or mineral can help to correct a medically confirmed deficiency, which may in turn make you feel better, but no multivitamin or vitamin or mineral supplement in itself can give you energy.

12

Fitness and Fun are not Mutually Exclusive

Exercise is almost as nasty as the word "diet" to some people. That's okay. I don't like the word diet. You don't have to like the word exercise. Call it something else. Call it your daily activity, or physical fitness, or playing, or getting off your butt! Call it anything you want. Just do it! Unless you have a medical condition that limits or prohibits daily exercise, it needs to be included in your daily life plan. Simply put, you must have some form of daily activity in order to get healthy. You don't have to go to all out extremes, but you do have to get moving. You don't have to buy all the latest fitness gear or join the most popular fitness club. All you really need is a good pair of tennis shoes and you are all set!

The easiest and best exercise to begin with if you are an exercise novice is pure and simple walking. Anyone can do it. It doesn't cost a thing and it doesn't take a heck of a lot of coordination! There are really no excuses not to do it. If walking is not your thing, then just find some activity that you enjoy doing. The point is to simply get moving. Cardiovascular exercises include any exercise that gets your heart pumping! A few suggestions include walking, hiking, running, biking, kick-boxing, aerobics, or dance.

Once you have your cardiovascular fitness routine in order, it is time to add some strength training sessions. You will need to include both cardiovascular and strength training exercises in your fitness plan. This does not have to become hours spent at the fitness club running on the treadmill or pumping iron. Thirty minutes of cardiovascular exercise at least 5 days a week and fifteen minutes of strength training every other day is all you need to get in and stay in shape. The key is you have to get moving somehow, some way every single day. No more couch potatoing every night with your best friend, Mr. Potato Chip. It doesn't matter when you exercise or what you do, just get up and do it! If the gym scene intimidates you, then do your own thing at home. And I don't buy the "I can't afford it" excuse. Save all your money from the soda and junk foods you won't be purchasing anymore, and go to the local discount store and buy yourself an exercise mat, a few hand weights, and a selection of exercise tapes that will start you on your way.

If you can't walk outside, and can't afford a gym membership, then save up for a treadmill, or an elliptical machine, or a stationary bike. And don't hang your laundry from it! Put your exercise equipment where you will use it daily. If your basement is not a place you hang out normally, then don't put it there. Place your equipment in a well-lit comfortable room where you want to hang out. I have my treadmill, free weights, exercise mat, and spinner bike proudly placed in what should be the breakfast sunroom. My room has all the amenities I need for a comfortable, fun work out. I have a ceiling fan and a floor fan, a television and a video tape player, and a compact disc player. I even have remote control and headphones for both the television and CD player so I won't bother other family members if I choose to exercise early in the morning. I have absolutely allowed myself no excuses for not working exercise into my daily life.

Some people work out better around others and need a fitness friend or need the stimulation of a gym. The secret is to find what you enjoy and stick with it. I don't always enjoy my work out. If I feel burned out, I take a day off. And I don't sweat it, because I know I will get back to it the next day. If I don't feel like running on my treadmill, I take a long walk with my dog. If I don't have time for a full session of weight training, I do a few push ups or floor exercises. The point is that I take the time to do something every day. It doesn't have to be a formal exercise routine; you just have to do something active. Exercise is like eating, it has to be a priority, but it need not be an obsession.

If you read about anyone that has made a commitment towards healthy living through changes in diet and lifestyle behaviors, you will notice a common thread among them all. They have all incorporated some kind of exercise into their daily lives. Most of them will have started with something simple like walking, before adding other physical activities into their lives. But once they catch the exercise bug, they all become addicted to a daily need to get up and move! And I am not talking about walking to the corner deli for your favorite ham and cheese sandwich. I'm talking about committing a specific amount of time to exercising and improving your fitness level.

I always tell my clients that you will never have successful, healthy, long-term weight management if you do not incorporate exercise into your daily life. I have had nutritional counseling sessions in which the entire appointment has been dedicated to discussing the client's exercise resistance and their willingness to find some type of activity that will work for them. If exercise becomes just another chore you have to do, you won't stick with it. If it works into your daily schedule fairly easily, and is an activity you really enjoy, then it becomes something you will look forward to.

Let me give you an example of one woman I counseled who had difficulty committing to daily exercise. Let's call this client Karla. Karla was a thirty-eight year old married, working mom with two daughters. She weighed 250 pounds when she first came into see me for weight management counseling. She was always well made up and neatly dressed. She was also motivated to get a hold of her life and make some changes to get healthy again. We had had several nutritional counseling sessions and Karla was making considerable changes in her nutritional habits, but it was time for her to focus on her exercise plan, which was nonexistent at best. She was trying to find time in her day to squeeze in exercise between work and the kids. We reviewed her day, hour by hour, to see where we might find some time. She had previously commented that she was a member at the local Y and had on occasion ridden the exercise bike there and always enjoyed this activity.

As we reviewed her day, we found a two-hour period of time after work and before she had to pick her daughters up from after-school activities. This was the time when she would normally go home and monge on just about anything she could put her hands on while she "destressed" from work. I asked her if that would be a good time for her to stop at the Y. Initially she was resistant to the idea. But I shot down each of her excuses. One of her biggest concerns was that she wouldn't have time to "clean up" before she picked up her daughters, and then she would be embarrassed in front of the other moms. I looked her straight in the eye and said, "Do you really think people are going to judge you harshly for coming to pick your girls up dressed in workout clothes with no make up on? And what do you care what other people think anyway? This is about you making positive changes for yourself. If you really want to know, those people will probably be thinking, 'Boy, am I jealous, Karla got to take time for herself and do something to make herself feel better, I sure wish I had the motivation to do that!'"

When Karla thought about the situation in a different light, she felt empowered and began her exercise routine. Before long she was a regular at the Y and she had even gotten her old bicycle out of the attic to ride outside when the weather cooperated. I am happy to report that after one year of nutritional counseling, Karla had lost more than sixty pounds and was a completely changed person, inside and out! She had caught the exercise bug!

Exercise and good nutritional habits go hand in hand. You cannot have one without the other. Making good nutrition and daily exercise a priority in your life will ensure you lifelong success with weight management.

13

Food Issues Specific to Women

As I have stated earlier, I wrote this book with the intention that it would benefit anyone willing to make the commitment towards healthy eating. But I would like to take a moment to address one specific group: women. Women are traditionally the caregivers, food gatherers, and food preparers in our society. There are exceptions to this rule, but in the majority of family units, it is the woman who assumes these roles. Therefore, I would like to focus specifically on moms.

In my nutritional counseling career, moms make up the majority of my client population. Moms these days have a hectic workload, regardless of whether they work outside the home or not. Most moms not only hold down part or full time jobs, but also do the majority of the housework, and they are responsible for a good portion of the daily kid care. Now I am not trying to pick on the dads here. I am simply presenting what is the norm in most family units. Or at least what the norm appears to be for many of my women clients. Many of the women who come to see me with weight control problems are just simply tired and frustrated in general with their busy, hectic lives. They are so overwhelmed with taking care of everything and everyone around them, that they have forgotten how to take care of themselves. Some call it "being a Mom." I call it "being a Martyr."

Most of these moms simply need to be told that it is okay and actually absolutely necessary for them to put themselves back up in number one position and take care of themselves. They have the mindset that if they do anything for themselves, then they are taking time away from their kids or their husbands or their other commitments. I spend quite a bit of time reassuring these women that they are not neglecting their "duties" by taking care of themselves. In fact, if they really want to be a good role model for their kids, they need to focus on doing just that. They need to take the time to get healthy, and in the process get happy and excited about their lives again. What a great gift to give your kids! A mom that doesn't have to be it all and do it all, but can be a good example to her children by being a well rounded, healthy individual who is able and willing to take care of herself. After all, in the end, isn't that exactly what we want for our children anyway?

Some of the women I see are new moms with babies and toddlers at home. Many, admittingly, have used their pregnancy as an excuse to "pig out," thinking that they will lose the weight easily when the baby finally comes. I can tell you from personal experience, they are in for a rude awakening! Losing those baby pounds can be quite difficult for a number of reasons. After the baby is born, weight loss will take a low priority on your "to do" list. New moms are tired and sleep-deprived. A state of being that I have come to find, may last my entire "mom-hood" career! Not only are new moms tired, but also hormones are in a state of turmoil those first few months after delivery. When you are tired from sleep deprivation, the last thing you want to think about is exercising. Instead, what do most tired people do to boost their energy level? They eat. When you are over-tired and sleep-deprived, you tend to crave simple sugars and of course caffeine to "wake yourself up." There is nothing like a sugar or caffeine buzz to make you feel more alive, even if it only lasts for a few minutes. But as I have described earlier, the sugar buzz won't last, you will be left just as tired as you were before eating that chocolate bar and worse, you will be left craving more simple carbohydrates. So what do you do to prevent all this? Easy! Just don't have kids! No, I'm only joking! What you can do starts from the first day you plan on getting pregnant or find out you are pregnant. That is the most critical time to be in the best nutritional shape you can possibly be in. Your doctor or a dietitian can guide you to the appropriate nutritional information that you should follow during your pregnancy. This information will tell you exactly how much weight is healthy for you to gain over the course of the pregnancy and which foods are best to include in your diet to provide adequate nutrients for your growing baby. Take these guidelines seriously and follow them like you have never followed a nutrition plan before! Whatever you do, don't use your pregnancy as an excuse to eat nightly banana splits and monge on junk food. I promise, you will pay the price in the long run.

On the flip side of the pregnancy weight gain issue; don't beat yourself up by feeling bad about having a few pounds to lose after the baby comes. If you are nursing, you will feel hungrier and need extra calories to support your breastfeeding. Now is not the time to diet and cut calories. Relax. Take it one step at a time, one day at a time. The best thing to do is to continue the healthy eating habits you have developed during the pregnancy. Give yourself a chance to recover, in body and soul! Follow your doctor's advice on when to add exercise back into your life. If you concentrate on eating healthy and living healthy and take the focus off your weight, you will find yourself getting back to the old you in no time at all.

All parents need to be cognizant of the fact that you will pass your food issues and your body image issues onto your children! It is so important for parents to get a hold of your own eating habits so that you can set a good example for your children. Most of us don't think twice about teaching our kids about good manners, proper etiquette, and good hygiene. But, teaching good nutritional habits and how to take care of our bodies from the inside out somehow gets pushed to the bottom of the "to do" list. Mothers, as the same sex parent, you are especially modeling behaviors for your daughters. Because of this modeling, it becomes even that much more important for you to be aware that your nutritional and exercise habits will influence your children.

14

Food is an Addictive Substance

I would like to discuss what I call "extreme food issues." This subject is near and dear to my heart because it involves the subject of eating disorders. People who suffer from eating disorders are most often grouped into two categories: anorexics, who use starvation to control their weight, and bulimics, who use bingeing and purging to control their weight. However, I would like to add a third category of food abusers: overeaters who don't purge and can't control their weight. All three disorders involve the abuse of food and the loss of control in one's life. I don't profess to be a psychologist with a fancy degree in food psychology and behavioral disorders. But, I have walked the walk and I can talk the talk when it comes to having lived life as an anorexic and having been fortunate to recover from a disorder that can eat at your heart and soul.

I could write an entire book on the emotional and control issues that feed into eating disorders, but for now I would simply like to address the idea of food as an abusive substance. Most people recognize alcohol and drugs (including cigarettes) as abusive substances. But few realize that food can also be an addictive, abusive substance. The main difference is that you can "quit" or "give up" the addictions to alcohol, drugs, or cigarettes. Granted, no addiction is easy to overcome, but you can live without alcohol or drugs. You cannot live without food. Therein lies the problem with this addiction.

I believe that we all have certain obsessive/compulsive tendencies. It is those tendencies that act as goal directors in most areas of our lives, helping us to be successful in our personal and professional lives. It is only when these obsessions and compulsions spin out of control that they cause problems. Simply put, this is what occurs in an eating disorder. A person uses food as their control lever. Anorexics and bulimics tend to get a more sympathetic ear because the general population perceives these disorders as "medical" conditions worthy of our empathy and support. On the other hand, the overweight, obese, and morbidly obese tend to get little sympathy and quite a bit of disdain from the "normal" weight community.

The irony of this situation is that all three eating behaviors are reflective of the same obsessive/compulsive/control disorder, but they are manifested in different ways. All three are acting out their obsessive/compulsive tendencies by using food as an addictive substance. The reasons why people fall into these food addictions are as varied as the individuals themselves. But I have discovered something from my personal experience with anorexia and from counseling people in nutrition: It is far more important to first make some of the lifestyle changes I have addressed in this book than it is to initially uncover the root of the problem. It is the old saying; which comes first, the chicken or the egg? This is not to imply that the underlying problems or events that initially triggered the eating disorder are not important or relevant. But generally, when a person starts making some real nutritional and lifestyle changes, these positive changes soon become new habits, and the person starts feeling better about, and in more control of, many aspects of their lives. This new feeling of confidence and control can then better enable a person to deal with the ghosts in the closets that may have led to the obsessive/compulsive/control issues in the first place.

15

Keeping Records and Keeping Life Simple

Your daily eating and exercise routine should be consistent and healthy, but that doesn't mean that these habits have to be time consuming or complicated. Let me reiterate one point: Food and exercise should be a priority in your life **not** an obsession.

The reason most diets fail is not because the person doesn't have the willpower or the wherewithal to follow the diet. It is simply that most diets are too complicated to be followed for any length of time. When I was in dietetics school, one of our class assignments was to follow a diet plan for the illness that we were studying at that particular time. One week our assignment was to follow a strict diabetic diet. We had to determine how many calories we could have each day. Next, we had to break down our daily meal plan into a certain percentage of carbohydrates, protein, and fat based on our daily calorie allotment. Then, we had to calculate the number of grams of each nutrient we were allowed to eat and spread those meals and snacks evenly throughout the day. Finally, we had to develop a weeklong menu that would fit that meal plan. Sound complicated? It was. Sound fun? It wasn't. It was impossible to calculate the protein, carbohydrate, and fat content in a serving of the mystery casserole in the dorm's cafeteria! When we reviewed our menus in the classroom, they were pathetic to say the least. We all had survived the week by eating simple non-combination foods like bread, peanut butter, and yogurt. Foods that actually had the nutritional breakdown in black and white on their respective labels.

That assignment was a huge eye opener for all of us. I walked out of that classroom realizing that any "diet" that expected you to follow specific guidelines for any period of time might be great in theory, but it was not realistic when applied to the real world. And after a few years of clinical practice, I also realized that simply convincing some of my cardiac rehab patients not to fry their hotdogs was a huge success! (Well, I was living in the Deep South at the time!)

Complicated diets don't work. Our lives are busy enough without having to worry about what percent of our calories should come from protein, fat, or carbohydrates and how to spread those calories perfectly throughout the day. Eating and food should be fun! A certain amount of planning and preparation is necessary, but healthy eating doesn't need to be complicated. You need to use some basic guidelines and a little common sense. Simplify your nutritional plan, and you will be successful in managing your weight.

Keeping a journal will help you improve your nutritional, exercise, and lifestyle habits. A common denominator in successful weight management is record keeping. Studies have proven that people are more likely to be successful with long-term weight loss goals if they keep a food diary. Recording what you eat keeps you honest. I encourage my clients to keep daily food intake records. You should record what you eat **immediately** after you eat it. If you wait until later in the day, you will forget about that handful of chocolate covered peanuts you ate after lunch. It is also helpful to record quantities of foods eaten. This does two things: It makes you realize just how out of whack your portion sizes may be, and it keeps you honest in the amount of hidden fat you may be using. Keeping accurate food records allows you to see where you may be having difficulties. Sometimes it is not what you are eating that is inappropriate, but how much of it you are eating. In addition to writing down what you eat and how much you eat, you will want to record when you eat. We are all creatures of habit. We tend to do similar things at similar times of the day. If you keep records, you can look back and see what your problem food patterns are. For example, you may record that every night while watching television you eat a bowl of ice cream. This is called habitual eating. You are not eating the ice cream because you are still hungry. You are not eating the ice cream because you are bored. Instead, eating a bowl of ice cream every night at 7:00 sharp has simply become a habit. Keeping a journal will help you pinpoint habitual eating so that you can change those habits that are sabotaging your weight loss efforts.

You may also want to record the emotions that you are feeling when you eat a particular food. You can make this as simple or complicated as you'd like. You can record that your stomach was growling, so you really were physiologically hungry. You can record that you were tired, sad, lonely, or that you were celebrating with friends. Keeping these records will help you tune into emotional eating habits. Recording your daily exercise is also helpful. Keeping track of your daily exercise holds you accountable, and helps you set and achieve your fitness goals.

Although record keeping is very helpful in the initial stages of making nutritional, fitness, and lifestyle changes, it does not have to be done forever. When you feel confident that you have made some permanent changes, you can relax in your record keeping. If you feel like you are getting off base in one area or another, you can go back to your journal and start recording your efforts again. I keep an ongoing record of my fitness routine on a calendar in my exercise room. I like to look back over my weekly exercise and see how many total miles I have run or how often I have done some weight training. It gives me a sense of accomplishment, and it helps me set new fitness goals when I'm feeling bored with my routine. When I feel that my eating habits have slipped, or that I need to get a better handle on my portion sizes, I write down my food intake for a day or two. Seeing what my food and fitness habits are in black and white always helps me to refocus my energies.

Often times I have clients who ask me for a preprinted food and exercise diary for them to keep their records in. I always say no. Why? Because, as I have said before, everyone is an individual and there is no one diet or exercise plan that works for everyone. Likewise, there is no one record keeping method that works for everyone. Those clients that are willing to keep food, exercise, and emotional diaries in their own individual ways will be the most successful in their efforts. I have had clients keep their records on loose-leaf notebook paper, in three ring binders, on laptop computers, or in teeny-tiny notebooks that they can keep in their purses or briefcases. When they take ownership of their records and create something that works for them as an individual, they are always more successful in their record keeping and in their eating, exercise, and lifestyle goals in general. It all goes back to what I said in the beginning of this book: I can give you the nutritional, exercise, and lifestyle suggestions to guide you down the path of successful weight management, but it is ultimately you who have to be willing to put the time, effort, and commitment into making the changes and individualizing the plan to fit your specific life situation.

16

Be Your Own Best Friend

This journey towards getting healthy and staying healthy can be kept simple, but it is not always easy. It is a journey that you will have to make for yourself and by yourself. You will have to be your own best friend and your own champion all along the way. This means not sabotaging yourself and not letting friends, coworkers, or family sabotage you or your efforts. That does not mean that you shouldn't have or accept help or support from others, only that you shouldn't rely on or expect that support.

Change is hard. Change is uncomfortable. People generally don't like change. If you are committed to changing your eating habits, your exercise habits, and your lifestyle habits, it is going to involve a lot of change. That change will be unnerving to you, and it will be unnerving to those around you.

I can remember when I first caught the "fitness bug." After my second child was born, I was feeling large and in charge! When my daughter was about three months old, I had a moment of clarity on a very sleep deprived day. I realized that the only way to start feeling better about myself was to get back to my old healthy eating habits and to add daily exercise to my life. I have never been a gym rat (I'm a little lacking in the aerobic/dance coordination department), and I didn't want to take too much time away from my children. Therefore, I realized that exercising at home would be the best option for me. After a little research, I decided to purchase an elliptical machine to use for my cardiovascular workout. I also purchased a simple floor mat, some hand weights, and a series of weight training tapes to improve my muscle strength. My initial goal was to workout on my elliptical machine for at least thirty minutes, five times a week, and to do at least one fifteen minute weight training tape three times a week. My husband helped me set up my exercise room, and he was pleased to see me excited about something since I had had some difficulty with post-partum baby blues.

Well, he was pleased until he realized how serious I was about changing my lifestyle. My lifestyle change meant he was going to have to do some changing as well, and he wasn't prepared for that. My thirty minutes of exercise had to fit into a very busy mom day. This meant getting up at 5:00 a.m. on some mornings to fit my exercise in before the kids woke up. Other days, it meant dad had to "parent" the kids while I had thirty minutes all to myself to exercise. It also meant that as my waistline slimmed down, his wasn't looking so trim! All of a sudden he wasn't as supportive of, or as happy for me, in the changes I had made. I got the guilt trip for not sleeping in with him on the weekends, or for waking him up with the noise from the elliptical machine, or for having him "parent" the kids when he wanted to play with his cars in the garage. I was being sabotaged by my best friend!

We finally had a heart to heart discussion about all of the changes I had made to improve my well being, and why he was no longer supporting my efforts. I would like to tell you that things improved from that moment on, but they didn't. It took time and it wasn't easy, but my husband learned to appreciate and to be proud of the changes I had made. And he loves to tell people that I am quite a sports anomaly: I am the most physically fit, yet athletically challenged person you could ever hope to meet! (He finds this fact quite amusing!) And in his own sweet time, my husband caught the fitness bug as well. He lost thirty pounds and now has a fancy road bike that he rides while pretending he's in the Tour de France! The point of this story is that I was fortunate that my husband decided to make eating, fitness, and lifestyle changes with me, because it was a lot more difficult, and not nearly as much fun, when I was doing it alone!

You will have similar challenges while changing your lifestyle. That friend you used to meet at the donut shop on Tuesday mornings isn't going to understand why you don't want to chat over coffee and pastries anymore. Your kids may whine and complain when you refuse to stop for fast food after soccer practice. Your coworkers may feel hurt and slighted when you don't join them munching on cookies in the staff break room. And your mate may entice you to sit down and watch television instead of going out for your daily walk.

Any number of these situations will occur as you go through the process of making life changes. And you will have to remain strong and confident and willing to stay the course to get past these challenges. It won't always be easy. It won't always be fun. It won't always be the popular thing to do. But it will be worth it in the long run.

17

Final Food for Thought

You may come to this final chapter and be wondering where are the lists of "good" foods and "bad" foods? Where is the meal plan? How many calories should you have every day? What should your maximum heart rate be to get the most out of your workout? Those are the kinds of questions that every other diet book attempts to answer. True to my word, this is a non-diet diet book.

I struggled with the notion of including specific meal plans with calorie guidelines and recipe suggestions. But I kept going back to the idea that every person is an individual with specific food preferences and life situations, not to mention varying degrees of culinary skills. I didn't want to have to assume that everyone knew how to cook or even liked to for that matter. But I do know that anyone can rip open a bag of lettuce, peel an orange, drink water, skip the junk food grocery aisle, and drive by the drive-bys! It is really that simple. And that brought me back to the goal of this book: to have people recognize that just making the simple changes I have outlined are enough to guarantee successful weight loss. You don't need specific calorie guidelines, menu plans, or fancy exercise routines to begin the process of healthy living. If you make all of the changes I have reviewed in the previous chapters regarding your eating, fitness, and lifestyle habits, you will be successful in managing your long-term weight goals. If you follow these guidelines, but find you want to kick it up a notch, you can find any number of novice to gourmet-style healthy cookbooks. Any cookbook endorsed by the American Dietetic Association or The American Heart Association is a sure winner. My personal favorite food magazine is *Cooking Light*. This magazine has recipes designed for both the seasoned cook as well as the culinary novice.

From the beginning, I made it clear that this would not be a book that would promise a quick fix, a magic pill, or tips on the latest fad diets. Anything you read or hear that promises you quick and easy weight loss is just an outright lie, no matter how much we all wish it were true. If those products, gimmicks, or diets were able to guarantee you safe, effective long-term weight loss in less time than it takes you to say the word "diet", then we would be a nation of very thin, very fit people. Instead, we are a nation struggling with an obesity crisis, always on the look out for a quick fix for our weight issues.

The mindset of many people seems to be that more is always better. This attitude flows over into many aspects of our lives—bigger food portions, bigger houses, bigger cars, and bigger vacations. I even see this attitude among the "fit" population. Some people who profess to be living a fit and healthy lifestyle are so obsessed with exercise that it consumes their lives. They aren't out enjoying the sunrise with a brisk morning walk. Instead, they focus on pushing themselves to their physical limits by training and running marathon after marathon. They aren't out enjoying the beauty of the countryside on a ten to thirty mile bike ride. Instead, their goal is to ride at least fifty miles at breakneck speed before they can even count it as a real workout. I am not trying to put down long distance endurance sports, but let's face it, we can't all be Lance Armstrong or Jackie Joyner-Kersee. My point is that just thirty minutes to an hour of moderate exercise every day is all you need to get fit and be healthy.

It is this extreme attitude that is not only affecting our eating and exercise habits, but seemingly every aspect of our lives. It has become an all-or-none mentality. The word "moderation" has been deleted from our vocabulary. For those of you who struggle with the notion of getting fit, eating right, and improving your health, it can be completely overwhelming and intimidating to try to keep up with this "extremist" mentality.

Instead of people getting excited about making exercise and good eating habits a part of their lives, some people are simply frustrated with the whole issue. So what do they do? They fall back into bad eating and lifestyle habits because it is what they know and it is comfortable. They opt to live in the opposite extreme of the "health nuts" by choosing a sedentary lifestyle with no food limits. What they fail to realize is that it is much more fun to relax and enjoy life with just a little bit of everything, instead of such an all-or-none approach. I for one am never giving up chocolate, but you won't find me eating an entire box of bonbons in one sitting either! Sometimes it is important to realize that less is more.

The less is more mentality is why I have attempted to keep this book short and sweet. Most of you reading this book have probably read volumes and volumes of weight loss tips and tried a million and one diets. My hope is that you take the positive, helpful guidelines you have learned in the past, add what you've learned from this book, and make a commitment towards a healthy, productive life. No more dieting, no more quick fixes, and no more living in an overweight body that you are miserable in.

If you keep things simple and moderate regarding eating and exercise, you will live a healthy life with long-term weight control. That is the quick fix, magic pill, and real deal. You can enjoy a life of good food and fun fitness, if you do so in moderation. If you overeat every day, you will be overweight. If you over exercise every day, you will wear out your joints and risk physical injury. If you overspend every day, you will deplete your bank account. It really is a simple concept. If you follow a moderately healthy eating and exercising lifestyle and keep your plan simple, you will be successful in your long-term weight management goals. You may still have other life issues, but they will be issues that you will now have the energy to deal with!

I hope that I have given you some food for thought.

0-595-30972-0